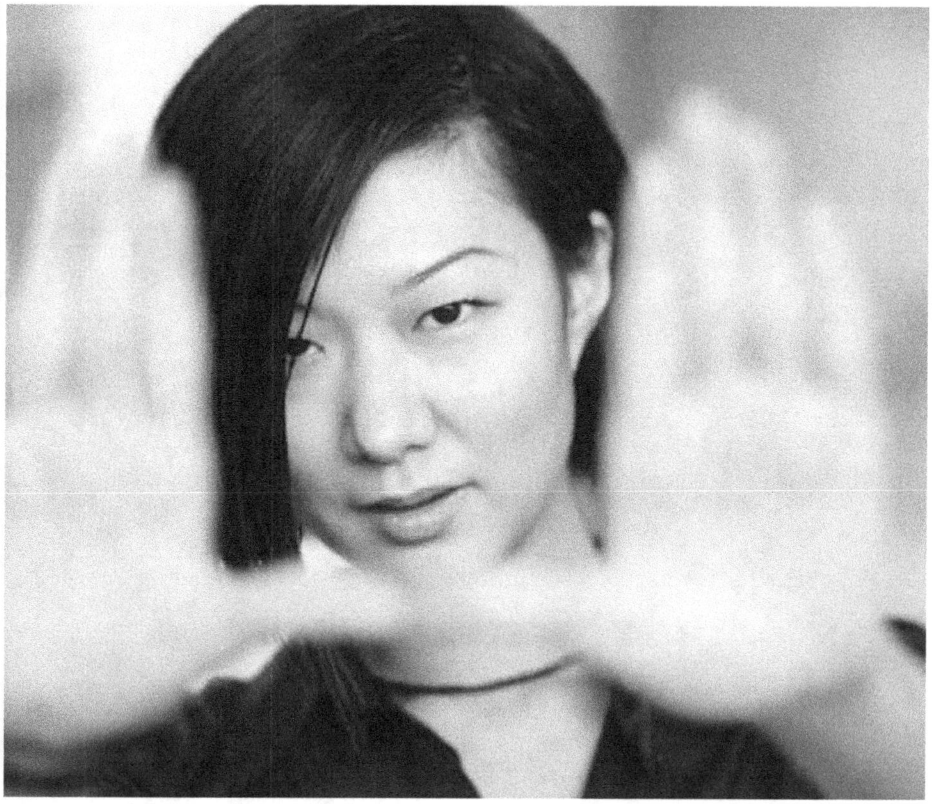

Adding Power to Our Voices

A Framing Guide for Communicating About Injury

CDC

Injury Prevention

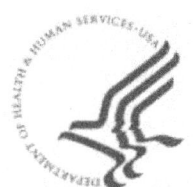

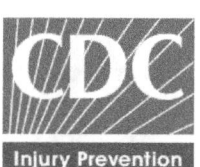

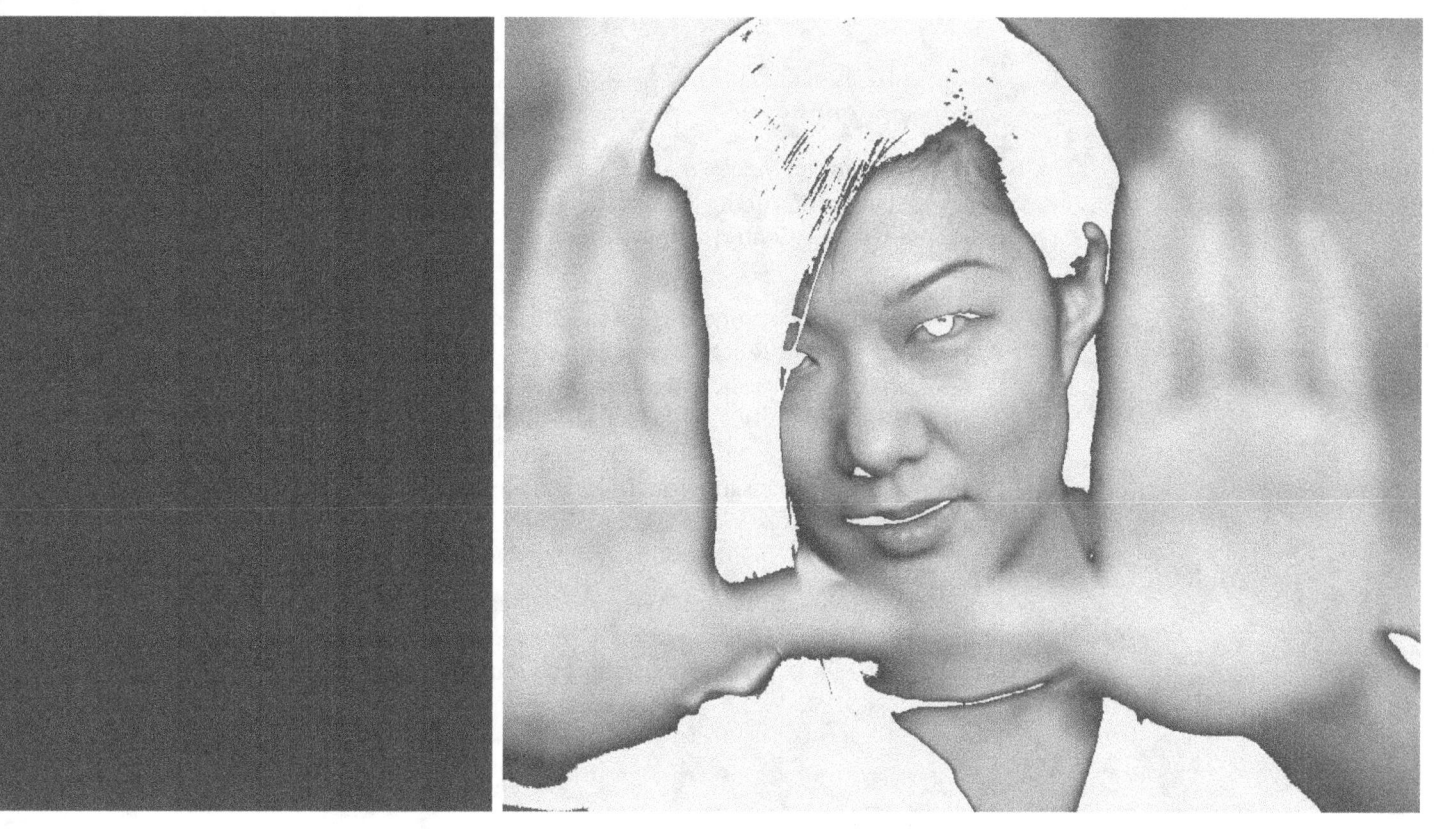

Adding Power to Our Voices
A Framing Guide for Communicating About Injury

National Center for Injury Prevention and Control
Atlanta, Georgia
2010
Version 2

Acknowledgments

Adding Power to Our Voices: A Framing Guide for Communicating About Injury is a publication of the National Center for Injury Prevention and Control, Centers for Disease Control and Prevention, U.S. Department of Health and Human Services

We acknowledge and appreciate the thoughtful contributions of our Expert Workgroup, including Robin Argue, Susan Gallagher, Andrea Gielen, Allison Lowe Huff, Angela Mickalide, Jim Hmurovich, Al Race, Ellen Schmidt, Eric Tash, and Elizabeth Wilson. We would also like to acknowledge the work of CDC staff who contributed to this document, including Teri Barber, Christy Cechman, Paige Cucchi, Leslie Dorigo, Susan Dugan, Emily Eisenberg, Kendra Godbold, Amy Harris, Gail Hayes, Wendy Heaps, Michele Huitric, Jennifer Middlebrooks, Jane Mitchko, Sara Schmit, Amanda Tarkington, and Marsha Vanderford.

Finally, thanks also go to Carol Freeman, Lucinda Austin, Marcia Cram, Joanne Milne, and Holly Reynolds Lee of ICF Macro and to their expert consultant, Susan D. Kirby, Ph.D., for assisting in the publication of this guide.

Suggested Citation: National Center for Injury Prevention and Control. *Adding Power to Our Voices: A Framing Guide for Communicating About Injury.* Atlanta, GA: US Department of Health and Human Services, Centers for Disease Control and Prevention; 2008 (revised March 2010). Available at: http://www.cdc.gov/injury.

Contents

Preface

When the CDC Injury Center asked communication professionals working in injury and violence prevention and response about their communication challenges, it became clear that messages about injury and violence need to reach and appeal to a broader audience to change public perceptions and have an influence on social and political will. Discussions with these professionals led to an effort to collaborate and coordinate messaging to achieve the greater goal of successfully elevating public awareness of injury and violence prevention and response.

Through formative research with the public, one societal value stood out as one that could speak to not only those with an existing interest or relationship with injury and violence prevention, but also could reach those who may have little previous exposure to the topic. This value that all could embrace — "We want a society where people can live to their full potential" — resonated with the public and injury communication professionals.

We took this information and created a guide that all injury and violence prevention and response professionals could use to develop messages that would benefit their injury-specific topic and the field as a whole. *Adding Power to Our Voices: A Framing Guide for Communicating About Injury* incorporates framing theory, message development techniques and vehicles for explaining public health statistics. When these tools are used to create messages for the public, your members or constituents, we anticipate these will prompt public interest and changes in perception and reaction to injury and violence prevention and response.

By using a common frame and coordinated messaging across injury materials and outreach activities, we give the whole injury field a boost whenever any specific injury issue is in the spotlight. It is our hope that, over time, our efforts to modify how we frame information about our field will change perceptions, and we will see a positive evolution in personal and societal consideration of injury and violence prevention and response.

Sincerely,
Ileana Arias, Ph.D.
Principal Deputy Director
Centers for Disease Control and Prevention

Adding Power to Our Voices: A Framing Guide for Communicating About Injury

We each work to address sometimes very different injury issues (prevention, response, violence, neglect, and unintentional injuries of all types). Yet, we all want to live in a society that believes and engages in injury and violence prevention and response initiatives that allow people to have the opportunity *to live to their full potential.*

Our mission at CDC's National Center for Injury Prevention and Control (CDC's Injury Center) is to prevent injuries and violence and reduce their consequences. *Adding Power to Our Voices* is designed to help organizations involved in injury and violence prevention and response speak with a consistent voice in building the social and political will needed to save lives and reduce injuries.

The purpose of this guide is to encourage the adoption and integration of a coordinated message strategy that is based on an overarching injury and violence prevention and response message frame and specific messages that link the injury or violence issue to the frame and are tailored to specific audiences. The guide provides framing and message development techniques and tools, including social math, to help injury and violence prevention and response programs create messaging that presents injury and violence in a way that reflects the broad and deeply held societal value of *living life to its full potential.* The coordinated message strategy can help us achieve a unified voice and increase the perceived value of injury and violence as an important public health problem, ultimately influencing the social and political will to lessen the burden of injury and violence.

> A coordinated message strategy can help change people's perceptions of the value of preventing and responding to injury and violence. This is critical to creating the social and political will to more fully support injury and violence prevention and response.

Common Communication Challenges

CDC's Injury Center invited input from a variety of injury communication professionals to explore our common communication challenges (See Table 1). These challenges represent significant hurdles for each of us in communicating about our individual injury issues. Not all challenges are felt equally given the diverse injury and violence prevention issues that we face. Those in the unintentional injury field grapple with the challenge of the belief that injuries are unpredictable or unavoidable while those in violence prevention encourage individual responsibility for the prevention of violence without blaming victims of violence. Yet, as we discovered in our conversations, these challenges can also help bind us together and provide a common foundation for collaboration.

This guide aims to help everyone involved in injury and violence prevention and response communicate in ways that build awareness that injuries and violence can be prevented and the consequences minimized when they occur.

The coordinated messaging tools in this guide can help to address many of the challenges that injury and violence prevention and response professionals have identified and build a strong infrastructure for injury communication that will last well into the future. The coordinated message strategy can help all injury and violence programs contribute to creating the change necessary to achieve the ambitious goal of a society where everyone can live to their full potential.

These challenges can help bind us together and provide a common foundation for collaboration.

Table 1. Injury Communication Challenges When Communicating With the Public
Injury and violence is seen as the responsibility of several fields (criminal justice, first responders, transportation, and education), which leads to the fracturing of the search for solutions.
Lack of understanding of the definition of injury and scope of the injury problem.
Lack of knowledge that solutions exist to reduce the impact of injury and violence.
Lack of individuals' sense of control over their risk environment (e.g., homes, workplaces, and schools).
Injury and violence is not understood as a public health issue.
Funding for injury programs is not commensurate with the magnitude of the problem.
Stigma associated with several types of injury such as sexual violence and suicide hampers open discussion.
Media coverage generally focuses on an individual event rather than the broader injury context.
Low levels of personal relevance or connections to injury.
Enduring beliefs of unintentional injury as unpredictable and not preventable.
Consequences of violence go beyond physical injury.

Leveraging Communication to Benefit All in the Injury Community

For this effort to succeed, we must build upon the existing communication work of all organizations working in injury and violence. We must engage those highly dedicated stakeholders, partners, volunteers, and staff members to continue to support their cause and be willing to connect their cause to the larger injury problem. Specific injury issues need to continue to thrive through tailored outreach that effectively reaches specific audiences.

Increasing understanding of injury and violence and the commitment to more fully address prevention and response can be accomplished by building on the hard-won visibility for specific injuries that has grown over the past few decades. Coordinated messaging is a foundation that can support and connect many different specific injury programs, while not taking anything away from each specific injury topic's unique messages.

Adding Power to Our Voices

The injury and violence field is small in comparison to other health fields. However, together we can have a louder voice than each can alone. Most stakeholders, especially the public, focus on one issue at a time (e.g., helping women, protecting children or fire safety). What if a brochure about older adult falls ends up in the hands of a traumatic brain injury prevention supporter? A coordinated message about how injury prevention, as a whole, can help people live to their full potential may give that supporter one more reason to support community programs that impact both traumatic brain injury and falls prevention. *By using a coordinated messaging strategy based on a common injury frame and supporting messaging across injury and violence materials and outreach activities, we give the whole injury field a boost whenever any specific injury issue is in the spotlight.*

The Bottom Line

If all injury and violence prevention and response programs adopt and integrate the coordinated message strategy, we can repeatedly convey the value-based full potential injury frame and specific injury and violence messages over time and across multiple outreach activities. As a result, the public can begin to better understand and value that preventing and responding to injuries can help people live to their full potential. This guide provides framing information and message development techniques, including social math, to help injury and violence programs and partners implement the coordinated communication strategy.

> If all injury programs convey the same value message of "full potential" over time and across multiple outreach activities, the public will come to understand and value the fact that preventing and responding to injuries can help people achieve their full potential.

Will You Add Your Voice?

Message Development—Coordinated Messaging

We can start to change public perceptions about injury and violence with the use of a coordinated message strategy. The strategy includes the integration of a broad overarching statement that expresses a core value held by many individuals in our society. We call this a concept frame. The concept frame can be adapted and integrated into injury and violence specific communication. This can be done by creating audience specific messages that link a specific injury or violence issue to the concept frame. The concept frame does not necessarily have to be the first statement you use. In fact, Injury Center supported focus groups show that audience response is greater when given dramatic statements up front to grab audience members' attention (See Appendix A). The use of a coordinated messaging strategy can be used with other communication techniques and approaches such as social marketing.

Making the Injury Issue Meaningful

Feedback from injury communication professionals and other research suggests that the public does not value injury and violence prevention and response as much as some other public health issues. Framing theory suggests that this difference may occur because the public and other audiences do not see how addressing injuries reflects their strongly held values or is a priority for achieving the kind of community they want to live in.

People's perceptions of an issue are created largely by what they already know and associate with that issue. This knowledge base has usually been cultivated over a long period of time through a variety of communication channels such as advertising, news media, TV, movies, word-of-mouth, internet, e-mails, and direct experience. These mental shortcuts, or dominant frames, allow individuals to quickly understand issues and interrelated facts. Many of the communication challenges we noted earlier represent dominant frames that make it difficult for individuals to hear and value messages about injury and violence prevention and response.

CDC's Injury Center used message framing theory and communication research to identify a core societal value that would change how people value preventing and responding to a wide range of injury and violence prevention issues. The research findings and consultation with partners indicate that the value of "we want a society where people can live to their full potential" is a frame that resonates across the spectrum of injury and violence issues.

> Research findings suggested the message frame, *"We want a society where people can live to their full potential"* received the most support overall as a strong cultural value statement.

Message Framing—How It Works

Message framing can help connect people to issues with a new perspective and establish new associations, thus changing the dominant frame. There are many facets to successfully framing an issue. Once identified, a new frame must be established through consistent, repetitive, strong, and broad-based communication, usually over a number of years. Linking an issue to a widely held core value helps start the framing process by resonating with the audience and increasing interest in learning more about how the issue connects with this core societal value.

Changing a Dominant Frame

A few decades back, the dominant frame in driving under the influence of alcohol or drugs might have included thoughts like, "It's those impaired drivers who have the problem." For a new frame, communication materials, tools, activities, and outreach would have to identify a new value statement that would make individuals think differently about driving under the influence and engage them to want to learn more and become involved. In the example of driving under the influence, the old dominant or concept frame of "we live in a society where individuals are responsible for their own actions" was changed over the years to "wanting to live in a society that cares about each other." In this case the frame was used to promote a program where friends share responsibility for preventing impaired driving. This new frame of caring and shared responsibility was communicated through TV show sitcoms, dramas, and even talk shows. Music and advertising reinforced the new frame. A more dominant message today is that "friends don't let friends drive drunk." It may seem daunting, but over time, with consistent and repetitive messaging, dominant frames can be changed for the better.

Applying the Message Frame

The remainder of this guide provides information and tools to help you craft injury specific messages that link your injury issue to the full potential frame. Tables 2 and 3 provide an example of coordinated messaging using the full potential frame. You can insert your specific injury into the text and adapt language to reflect how your injury issue and work in injury and violence prevention and response best connects with the overarching frame of wanting all individuals to live to their full potential. The Injury Framing Tool on page 19 provides a template for applying the full potential frame, while pages 14-16 provide message development techniques, including social math, to help you create messages that will resonate with your intended audiences. For additional examples of framing in use, visit the Injury Framing Collaborative Workspace: http://www.injuryframing.safestates.org. The Injury Framing Collaborative Space is a tool for professionals working in injury and violence prevention and response to share materials, resources, and best practices relating to injury framing.

CDC's Injury Center is using the "full potential" frame in its communication. For example, the frame was incorporated into fall prevention communication and appears on the CDC website (http://www.cdc.gov/ncipc/preventingfalls).

We want a society where older adults can live to their full potential. While falls are a threat to the health and independence of older adults and can significantly limit their ability to remain self-sufficient, the opportunity to reduce falls among older adults has never been better. Today, there are proven interventions that can reduce falls and help older adults live better and longer.

Table 2. "Full Potential" Message Concept	
Concept Frame (Societal Value)	We want a society where people can live to their full potential.
Short Expression:	Organizations, communities, and individuals should work together to help all Americans live healthier, more productive lives. We can take steps to lower the risk of injuries and violence and help those who are injured achieve full recovery.
Sample "Elevator Speech"*:	My organization is part of a movement to reduce the risk of injuries and improve the immediate response to those who are injured so that everyone can live his or her life to their full potential. Each year, injuries resulting from a wide variety of physical and emotional causes—including motor vehicle crashes, sports trauma, violence, [insert injury] or neglect—keep millions of adults and children from achieving their goals and making the most of their talents and abilities. But thanks to the discoveries of science and injury research, there are steps that [communities and individuals] can take—including [specific program(s)]—that can stop injuries before they happen and increase the likelihood for full recovery when they do. By incorporating these strategies into the community and everyday activities, we can improve the opportunity for all individuals to lead active, useful, and fulfilling lives.
Sample Press Release Copy:	Injuries and violence are a significant and largely preventable problem. Injury prevention research has provided new information and new tools to address this problem and help millions of people live to their fullest potential. Many of the injuries that keep adults and children from enjoying fulfilling, productive lives—such as [specific injuries]—can be prevented using known prevention measures—including [specific injury programs]. When injuries occur, chances for a full recovery can be improved with specialized emergency care, such as [specific injury program]. Organizations, communities, and individuals should work together in a coordinated effort to promote and adopt these kinds of programs to ensure that every person enjoys the highest possible quality of life.

*An elevator speech is an overview of an idea for a product, service, or project. The name reflects the fact that an elevator pitch can be delivered in the time span of an elevator ride (say, 30 seconds or 100 to 150 words).

A Tailored Message for Organizations Involved in Violence Prevention

CDC's Injury Center understands the difficulty in developing coordinated messaging that encompasses the broad spectrum of injury issues and that will resonate with people who work daily to alleviate the suffering caused by those injuries. Through our research, individuals involved with violence prevention expressed the importance of a message that also contained the concept of *freedom from fear* of violence. Participants across the spectrum of injury also liked the firm and direct statement that, *"Injuries and violence are significant and largely preventable,"* because the statement is clear and because injuries and violence are not 100 percent preventable. Table 3 presents some additional message points for violence prevention.

Table 3. Additional Message Points for Organizations in Violence Prevention	
Concept Frame (Societal Value):	We want a society where people can live to their full potential.
Sample Press Release Copy:	In order for adults and children to realize their full potential, they must have safe places to live, work, and play where they can enjoy every aspect of their lives without worry about violence or injury. Programs that use the science of injury prevention to reduce the risk of violence, injury, and their associated consequences are available—including [specific programs]. When individuals and communities join forces with business and government to implement these violence prevention measures, we can help people live fulfilling lives, safe from hurt and harm.

Framing Tools

Message Development Considerations

Integrating coordinated messaging into your communication materials is easier than you might think. First, consider the full potential injury frame and then create messages that link your specific injury issue to the frame. The following message development considerations will help you create messages that have a greater impact with your intended audience. The considerations were identified through research with the public.[1,2]

1. Make a strong and dramatic statement about the injury problem.

    a. "Injuries are the leading cause of death in the first four decades of life, but they don't have to be—many injuries are preventable."

2. Include lists of a wide range of injuries that might seem unrelated to your specific injury issue, but can help frame the injury field as one field. This approach will also help audiences understand which specific types of health problems fit under the umbrella we call "injury."

    a. "Injuries result from a wide variety of physical and emotional causes—including motor vehicle crashes, sports trauma, violence, or neglect."

3. Use positive, action-oriented statements to present solutions early in the message.

    a. "There are steps that communities and individuals can take that are proven to stop injuries before they happen."

    b. "Injury and violence prevention research has provided new information and new tools to address this problem."

4. Use inserts of specific injury issues and programs to customize the message to your injury area.

    a. "Many of the injuries that keep adults and children from enjoying fulfilling, productive lives—including [specific injuries]—can be avoided or reduced by using prevention measures—including [specific injury programs]."

    b. "When injuries occur, chances for a full recovery can be improved with specialized emergency care, such as [specific injury program]."

[1] National Center for Injury Prevention and Control. (2007). *Executive summary of audience research recommendations for coordinated communication message frame and dissemination.* Centers for Disease Control and Prevention, U.S. Department of Health and Human Services, Atlanta, GA.

[2] Austin, L., Mitchko, J., Freeman, C., Kirby, S., & Milne, J. (2009). Using framing theory to unite the field of injury and violence prevention and response: "Adding Power to Our Voices." *Social Marketing Quarterly, 15(S1)*, 35-54.

5. Highlight the value of personal responsibility and community action—characterize organizations as partners.

    a. "Individuals can live healthier, more fulfilling lives by taking steps to protect themselves from injuries and prevent violence from occurring."

    b. "When individuals and communities join forces with business and government to implement these prevention measures, we can help people live fulfilling lives, safe from hurt and harm."

6. Reinforce the science of injury and violence prevention (without the use of jargon).

    a. "Thanks to the discoveries of science and injury and violence research, there are steps that communities and individuals can take."

    b. "Injury and violence prevention research has provided new information and new tools to address this problem."

7. Ensure that the message includes an "ask" or call to action.

    a. "Organizations, communities, and individuals can work together in a coordinated effort to promote and adopt these kinds of programs to ensure that every person enjoys the highest possible quality of life."

8. End by reinforcing the value message and reminding individuals that the actions they take can help achieve the value message (full potential) and create the kind of world that they want. This reinforcement of the value message is critical.

    a. "When individuals and communities join forces with business and government to implement these violence prevention measures, we can help people live fulfilling lives, safe from hurt and harm."

9. Remember that this work is designed to help create the social and political will to address injury and violence prevention through the socio-ecological model[2]. Sometimes different elements of the social ecology will be the focus of our messages to build awareness of and desire for solutions to injury and violence issues. While it may be appropriate to focus messages on what individuals can do to protect themselves from unintentional injuries (e.g., use of safety belts), violence prevention requires greater focus on individual responsibility for refraining from violence and on community-level change. We must ensure that our messages do not have the unintended consequence of implying that victims of violence are to blame.

CDC uses a four-level **social-ecological model** to better understand injury and violence and the effect of potential prevention strategies. This model considers the complex interplay between individual, relationship, community, and societal factors. It allows us to address the factors that put people at risk for experiencing or perpetrating injuries and violence.

10. Words of caution when integrating coordinated messaging:

    a. Frame preventive and response actions as giving people more freedom to live to their full potential because they will be injury-free and able to pursue their goals.

    b. Do not dwell on the injury problem and provide exhaustive lists of the statistics of the problem. People want to know about solutions, how they will be accomplished, and what they will cost.

    c. Do not describe injury problems using a single situation (e.g., a specific child abuse case). Instead, describe the context around how injury and violence happens over the long term and not as a single event.

Social Math and Framing[3]

Social math is "the practice of translating statistics and other data so they become meaningful to the audience"[4]—it makes the statistics and numbers surrounding an issue meaningful to people by vividly communicating those numbers. When combined with other frame elements, social math is a tool that can help guide people to think about the social and built environments surrounding the behavioral choices that individuals make. Social math helps messages resonate with the target audience by referencing or comparing the issue numbers to:

◆ Familiar numbers or costs (e.g., cost of car payment)

◆ Dramatic events (e.g., the number of residents displaced following Hurricane Katrina)

◆ Costs that are smaller and understandable (e.g., the program would cost less than the cost of a cup of coffee each day)

◆ Current numbers from other issues (e.g., it's more than one-third of what we spend on prescription medication each year).

As an example, a message can state that over 1.6 million people experience a traumatic brain injury each year. That is pretty abstract and gives the reader no comparison to things they know and understand in daily life. But if the message states that more people experience a brain injury each year than can fill Boston Red Sox' Fenway Park 35 times, the reader then has some visual cue and dramatic reminder of the size of the problem. Without using social math, communicators will try to convey a lot of abstract numbers to people who are already overloaded with information.

3, 4 Dorfman, L., Woodruff, K., Herbert, K., & Ervice, J. (2004). *Making the case for early care and education: A message development guide for advocates* (pp. 112-114). Berkeley, CA: Berkeley Media Studies Group. Available at www.bmsg.org/documents/YellowBookrev.pdf.

Social math helps audiences remember important facts and helps those facts become more salient. When using social math, it is critical to select a social math fact that is 100 percent accurate, visual if possible, dramatic, and appropriate for the target audience. Using a baseball social math fact for a target audience that does not know about or connect with baseball would be ineffective. Appendix B of this guide provides more information on using social math as well as additional examples.

Injury Framing Tool

The Injury Framing Tool is intended to help you apply a coordinated message strategy to your own injury or violence issues. The tool is designed to help you create effective messages that link to the injury frame *"We want a society where people can live to their full potential."* These messages can then be integrated into all of your communications (e.g., websites, fact sheets, publications, and press releases). Before you begin to craft your injury or violence specific messages, you need to identify your intended audience, that is, who you want to reach and influence with your communications.

Effective messages should be tailored to your audience. To help tailor your messages, you should consider your audience's current knowledge, attitudes, and behaviors relating to your injury issue. You can gather information about your audience through secondary data collection (literature reviews, existing studies) or primary data collection (interviews, focus groups, and surveys). If possible, you should test your frame-based messages with members of your target audience. Refer to Formative Research Appendix C for additional information. We encourage you to create messages for your injury or violence issue and organization and share your work with others in the field. You can share examples of your work with other injury and violence professionals using the Injury Framing Collaborative Space: http://www.injuryframing.safestates.org.

Using the Injury Framing Tool:

The Injury Framing Tool is divided into three sections:

What Broad Statement Can You Make To Link Your Injury Issue to the Full Potential Frame and the Coordinated Message Strategy?

◆ This section is designed to help you develop statements or messages that link your specific injury or violence issue to the societal value of believing that everyone should have the opportunity to achieve their full potential. You should develop injury or violence specific messages linking to the full potential frame for each audience you intend to reach. The message development techniques on pages 14-16 can help you craft messages that will resonate with your target audiences.

Social Math Examples

- Every 35 minutes an older adult dies from a fall-related injury.

- Nationwide implementation of effective school-based programs to prevent youth violence could result in 187,000 fewer fight-related injuries among high school students. That's equivalent to nearly 7,500 classrooms of students.

What Do You Want to Say About Your Injury Issue?

◆ This section is designed to help you communicate the size and scope of your injury or violence issue and its influence on your audience's lives. This is where social math comes into play. Refer to pages 33-39 for social math tips.

What Action Do You Want to Tell Your Audience to Take?

◆ This section offers specific recommendations and protective actions one can take to prevent injuries and violence. This is your call to action. To change the frame of injury, we must change the way the public considers their participation in preventing injuries. Although not all injuries are preventable or predictable, many can be influenced by policies, community initiatives, and personal and societal responsibility.

Pulling It All Together

◆ This section will help you write your final message once you've identified all your message components. Refer to the message development tools in the Framing Guide to help you create the most effective messages.

Following the Injury Framing Tool template, you will find examples for various injury and violence prevention and response issues.[5]

---

[5] The examples provided in this section are for illustrative purposes only. The messages have not been tested with members of the intended audience.

Injury Framing Tool

This tool is designed to help you create effective messages that incorporate the message development strategies in the Framing Guide and link your injury issue to the overarching injury frame:

We want a society where people can live to their full potential.

Injury Issue: _____

Intended Audience: _____

Intended Outcome (Communication Goal): _____

What broad statement can you make to link your injury issue to the full potential frame and the coordinated message strategy?

- For each of your audiences, what message will link or associate your specific injury issue to the injury field as a whole and to the idea that injuries and violence can be prevented?

- What can you say that will link your injury issue to the societal value of believing everyone should have the opportunity to achieve their full potential?

Write your linking statement(s) below. Refer to additional message development techniques in the Framing Guide.

What do you want to say about your injury issue?

- How can you help your audience understand the size and scope of your injury issue?
- How can your translate your statistics and data so they are interesting and meaningful to your audience? What social math examples can you use? (Refer to the social math section of the Framing Guide for social math tips.)
- What can you say that will describe your specific programs or activities as a way to address the injury issue (as a solution to the problem)? What is the science or evidence base for the programs/activities suggested?

Write your statements and social math facts below.

What action do you want your audience to take?

- What actions do you suggest that your audience take relating to your specific program or activity?
- If focused on individual behavior change, what do you want your audience to know they can do to protect themselves?
- What is your call to action?

Write your action-oriented statements below.

Pulling It All Together

- Now that you've identified the message components above, it's time to create a message that will move your audience to action. The message development tools in the Framing Guide can guide you in creating the most effective message for your audience.

Write your final message below.

Injury Framing Tool Example

This tool is designed to help you create effective messages that incorporate the message development strategies in the Framing Guide and link your injury issue to the overarching injury frame:

We want a society where people can live to their full potential.

Injury Issue: Child Maltreatment

Intended Audience: Community Based Organizations

Intended Outcome (Communication Goal): Increase support at the community level for programs and policies that promote positive parent child interactions

---

What broad statement can you make to link your injury issue to the full potential frame and the coordinated message strategy?

- For each of your audiences, what message will link or associate your specific injury issue to the injury field as a whole and to the idea that injuries and violence can be prevented?
- What can you say that will link your injury issue to the societal value of believing everyone should have the opportunity to achieve their full potential?

Write your linking statement(s) below. Refer to additional message development techniques in the Framing Guide.

- Injuries and violence are significant and largely preventable public health problems.
- We all want a community where people, especially our children, can live to their full potential.
- Child abuse and neglect is a substantial public health issue with short- and long-term negative effects on health and behavior.
- Research shows us healthy relationships act as a buffer against harmful childhood experiences.

What do you want to say about your injury issue?

- How can you help your audience understand the size and scope of your injury issue?
- How can your translate your statistics and data so they are interesting and meaningful to your audience? What social math examples can you use? (Refer to the social math section of the Framing Guide for social math tips.)
- What can you say that will describe your specific programs or activities as a way to address the injury issue (as a solution to the problem)? What is the science or evidence base for the programs/activities suggested?

Write your statements and social math facts below.

- Children who are abused or neglected are at a higher risk for health problems as adults, including alcoholism, smoking, suicide, and certain chronic illnesses, as well as aggressive behavior, adolescent delinquency, adult criminality, and the transgenerational perpetration of abuse and neglect.

- In 2008, Child Protective Services confirmed 905,000 cases of child abuse and neglect. Confirmed cases are considered only a fraction of the problem, yet this number is still greater than the entire population of Delaware.

- Evidence based prevention programs and policies that encourage and promote positive parent interactions and improve parenting skills can provide parents and caregivers with the skills they need to better manage behavior before abuse or neglect can occur.

What action do you want your audience to take?

- What actions do you suggest that your audience take relating to your specific program or activity?
- If focused on individual behavior change, what do you want your audience to know they can do to protect themselves?
- What is your call to action?

Write your action-oriented statements below.

- As community based organizations, you can ensure that young people in your area live healthier more fulfilling lives by supporting programs and policies that help parents enhance their ability to foster safe, stable, and nurturing relationship with their children.

- Every community can take steps to help assure safe, stable, and nurturing relationships for children. The costs are small compared with the benefits that can be realized in dollars saved, in the revitalized lives children can live now, and in the contributions these young people can make in the future.

Pulling It All Together

- Now that you've identified the message components above, it's time to create a message that will move your audience to action. The message development tools in the Framing Guide can guide you in creating the most effective message for your audience.

Write your final message below.

Imagine the impact on society if every person in the State of Delaware experienced problems such as alcoholism, smoking, suicide, certain chronic illnesses, aggression, and violent behavior. Fortunately, this isn't a real life scenario, but it could be. Children who are abused or neglected are at a high risk of developing just such problems, and last year's confirmed cases of child abuse and neglect topped 905,000—a number greater than the population of Delaware.

Thanks to research on injury and violence prevention, we know there are proven steps that communities and individuals can take before abuse or neglect can occur. In fact, evidence-based prevention programs and policies that encourage and promote positive parent interactions and enhance parenting skills can provide parents with the skills they need to better manage behavior.

As community based organizations, you can ensure that children in your community live healthier more fulfilling lives by supporting programs that help parents become better parents. Encourage widespread adoption of evidence-based prevention strategies. Every community can take steps to help assure safe, stable, and nurturing relationships for children. The costs are small compared with the benefits that can be realized in dollars saved, in the enhanced lives children can live now, and in the contributions these young people can make in the future.

Injury Framing Tool Example

This tool is designed to help you create effective messages that incorporate the message development strategies in the Framing Guide and link your injury issue to the overarching injury frame:

We want a society where people can live to their full potential.

Injury Issue: <u>Older Adult Falls</u>

Intended Audience: <u>Older Adults</u>

Intended Outcome (Communication Goal): <u>Reduce older adult falls by teaching prevention techniques</u>

What broad statement can you make to link your injury issue to the full potential frame and the coordinated message strategy?

- For each of your audiences, what message will link or associate your specific injury issue to the injury field as a whole and to the idea that injuries and violence can be prevented?
- What can you say that will link your injury issue to the societal value of believing everyone should have the opportunity to achieve their full potential?

Write your linking statement(s) below. Refer to additional message development techniques in the Framing Guide.

- Injuries and violence—including injuries to older adults from fires, motor vehicle crashes, and falls—are significant and largely preventable.
- Thanks to research, we know we can take actions to prevent injuries and premature deaths from falls.
- Preventing falls from happening in the first place can help older adults live longer and enjoy a better quality of life.

What do you want to say about your injury issue?

- How can you help your audience understand the size and scope of your injury issue?
- How can your translate your statistics and data so they are interesting and meaningful to your audience? What social math examples can you use? (Refer to the social math section of the Framing Guide for social math tips.)
- What can you say that will describe your specific programs or activities as a way to address the injury issue (as a solution to the problem)? What is the science or evidence base for the programs/activities suggested?

Write your statements and social math facts below.

- Each year almost 2.1 million older Americans are seen in emergency departments for falls. If instead these older adults were practicing Tai Chi or taking exercise classes, they would fill more than 140,000 classrooms.
- Every 35 minutes an older adult dies from a fall-related injury.
- Many of the injuries caused by falls that keep older adults from enjoying healthy and independent lives can be avoided by prevention measures such as exercise, vision correction, and medication adjustment.
- These proven steps can help reduce health care costs and greatly improve older adults' quality of life.

What action do you want your audience to take?

- What actions do you suggest that your audience take relating to your specific program or activity?
- If focused on individual behavior change, what do you want your audience to know they can do to protect themselves?
- What is your call to action?

Write your action-oriented statements below.

- As an older adult, you can help prevent falls by exercising, talking to your doctor or pharmacist about your medications, and ensuring your vision is properly corrected.
- Talk to your doctor to make sure it's safe for you to take an exercise class.
- For more information, visit the CDC website at www.cdc.gov/injury.

Pulling It All Together

- Now that you've identified the message components above, it's time to create a message that will move your audience to action. The message development tools in the Framing Guide can guide you in creating the most effective message for your audience.

Write your final message below.

Every 35 minutes an older adult dies from a fall related injury. But the fact is, many of the injuries that keep older adults from enjoying fulfilling, productive lives—motor vehicle crashes, fires and, yes, falls—can be avoided.

Thanks to research, we now know that you can lower your chance of falling by exercising, making proper medication adjustments, and ensuring your vision is properly corrected. These simple steps can help save health care costs and greatly improve your quality of life.

So make an appointment with your doctor to review your medication, check your vision, and ask what types of exercise are best for you. Falling isn't a natural part of getting older. You can take control of your quality of life by taking these simple steps to prevent falls.

For more information, visit the CDC website at www.cdc.gov/injury.

Injury Framing Tool Example

This tool is designed to help you create effective messages that incorporate the message development strategies in the Framing Guide and link your injury issue to the overarching injury frame:

We want a society where people can live to their full potential.

Injury Issue: Traumatic Brain Injury from sports and recreation-related activities

Intended Audience: Family members of people who ride bicycles and/or participate in other sports and recreational activities

Intended Outcome (Communication Goal): Decrease the incidence of injury by increasing usage of bicycle helmets and other protective sports equipment. that promote positive parent child interactions

---

What broad statement can you make to link your injury issue to the full potential frame and the coordinated message strategy?

- For each of your audiences, what message will link or associate your specific injury issue to the injury field as a whole and to the idea that injuries and violence can be prevented?

- What can you say that will link your injury issue to the societal value of believing everyone should have the opportunity to achieve their full potential?

Write your linking statement(s) below. Refer to additional message development techniques in the Framing Guide.

- Injuries and violence are a significant and largely preventable public health problem.

- Thanks to a range of injury and violence prevention work that is taking place today, Americans are more able to reach their full potential in the world.

- By taking steps to prevent injuries that might result from a wide variety of causes—including motor vehicle crashes and collisions or falls during bike riding or sports activities—we can all live healthier and more fulfilling lives.

What do you want to say about your injury issue?

- How can you help your audience understand the size and scope of your injury issue?
- How can your translate your statistics and data so they are interesting and meaningful to your audience? What social math examples can you use? (Refer to the social math section of the Framing Guide for social math tips.)
- What can you say that will describe your specific programs or activities as a way to address the injury issue (as a solution to the problem)? What is the science or evidence base for the programs/activities suggested?

Write your statements and social math facts below.

- More than 200,000 people visit U.S. emergency departments each year for sports and recreation-related traumatic brain injuries—that's enough to fill the 2010 Super Bowl stadium close to 3 times. And these don't include participants who are seen by other health care providers outside of the emergency department.
- With the findings from scientific research, we know that bicycle helmets and other sports helmets can prevent or reduce the severity of brain injuries.

What action do you want your audience to take?

- What actions do you suggest that your audience take relating to your specific program or activity?
- If focused on individual behavior change, what do you want your audience to know they can do to protect themselves?
- What is your call to action?

Write your action-oriented statements below.

- You can help ensure that the ones you love have every opportunity to lead active, fulfilling lives—encourage your loved ones to use a properly fitted helmet and other appropriate protective gear every time they ride a bike or participate in sports where helmets are recommended.
- To find out more information on preventing this and other injuries, visit www.cdc.gov/injury.

Pulling It All Together

- Now that you've identified the message components above, it's time to create a message that will move your audience to action. The message development tools in the Framing Guide can guide you in creating the most effective message for your audience.

Write your final message below.

Each year more than 200,000 people are treated in U.S. emergency departments each year for sports- and recreation-related traumatic brain injuries. That's enough people to fill the 2010 Super Bowl stadium close to 3 times. This doesn't mean we need to stop being active, though.

By taking steps to prevent injuries that might result from a wide variety of causes—including collisions or falls during bike riding or sports activities—we can all live life to its full potential. With the discoveries of scientific research, we know that wearing a bicycle helmet and other sports helmets can prevent or reduce the severity of brain injuries.

You can help ensure that the ones you love have every opportunity to lead active, fulfilling lives. Encourage your loved ones to use a properly fitted helmet or other protective gear every time they ride a bike or participate in sports where helmets are recommended. To find out more information about preventing sports and recreation-related brain injuries, visit http://www.cdc.gov/TraumaticBrainInjury.

Our Call to Action

The public sees and hears a variety of safety, health, and wellness messages every day. Still, many members of the public do not believe that injuries and violence are preventable if individuals and communities work together. Table 1 on page 8 highlights some of the communication challenges of the injury and violence prevention field. By addressing the challenges through a coordinated frame, we help the injury field as a whole, and, when our overarching injury and violence prevention and response messages get through to a wider audience, we all benefit. The public becomes more aware of all that is "injury," the injury field gains more visibility, and *we all benefit from positive responses that lead us toward living our lives to the fullest potential.*

To accomplish this vision and have a widespread impact, we need to take these actions:

◆ Adopt and integrate the full potential frame into our injury specific communication,

◆ Develop and use messages that link our specific injury issues to the full potential frame, and

◆ Repeat our specific injury messages across all injury areas, channels, and audiences.

Let's add power to our voices by using the framing approach.

Appendix A

NCIPC Coordinated Injury Communication: Message Frame Testing Executive Summary[6]

The Centers for Disease Control and Prevention's National Center for Injury Prevention and Control and ICF Macro conducted message testing research through in-depth policymaker interviews and focus groups with the general public. Research explored NCIPC's "full potential" concept frame and other message characteristics that could be used for coordinated communication about injury and violence prevention and response. A concept frame, as identified in CDC's framing guide, Adding Power to Our Voices, is a "broad overarching statement expressing a core value held by many individuals in our society" (p. 10).[7]

Injury areas identified as NCIPC priorities included:

◆ Child maltreatment

◆ Older adult fall prevention

◆ Traumatic brain injury (TBI).

Research at a Glance		
Participants	Injury-Specific Messages	Methods
Older adults 65+	Older adult falls	4 online/telephone focus groups (5-7 participants each)
Parents of youth under 18	Child maltreatment	4 online/telephone focus groups (5-7 participants each)
Both older adults 65+ and parents of youth under 18	TBI	4 online/telephone focus groups (5-7 participants each)
State-level policymakers	Older adult falls Child maltreatment TBI	7 phone interviews (randomly selected injury topics)

Research Questions

1. How is the injury frame of "living to one's full potential" perceived by the public and policymakers?

2. How can specific injury messages be crafted using the injury frame to contribute to the public and policymakers' understanding of injury issues and motivate them to take action?

Additional research question to assist the Division of Violence Prevention:

3. How can research on the "full potential" frame also inform the Division of Violence Prevention's efforts to communicate about "safe, stable, and nurturing relationships" (SSNRs)?

[6] National Center for Injury Prevention and Control. (2009). *NCIPC Coordinated Injury Communication: Message frame testing research report.* Centers for Disease Control and Prevention, U.S. Department of Health and Human Services, Atlanta, GA.

[7] National Center for Injury Prevention and Control. (2008). *Adding Power to Our Voices: A Framing Guide for Communicating About Injury.* Centers for Disease Control and Prevention, U.S. Department of Health and Human Services, Atlanta, GA.

Methods

Twelve online/telephone, 90-minute focus groups (5 to 7 members each, 66 participants total) were
conducted with:

1. Older adults ages 65+
2. Parents of youth under age 18.

Seven in-depth, 30-minute phone interviews were conducted with state-level policymakers. Each focus group and interview participant received a message on the "full potential" concept and two messages on a specific injury (see chart on right).

Findings and Recommendations

Research findings were compared to findings in the earlier phase of research and the coordinated messaging concepts in the Adding Power to Our Voices framing guide.

Findings were similar to previous findings and recommendations in the framing guide in that:

◆ Participants identified with the "full potential" concept frame.

◆ Participants liked the social math examples, especially those that they could strongly identify with, and they wanted to see this information early on in the message.

◆ Participants preferred strong and dramatic statements about the injury problem.

◆ Participants liked concise and action-oriented messages with a clear call to action.

◆ Participants liked positive messages that described tangible benefits to them.

◆ Participants wanted specific injury information customized to one specific injury area.

◆ Participants liked the focus on community action and needed more reinforcement about the responsibility for injury and violence prevention and response.

◆ Participants, particularly policymakers, wanted science-driven information.

In a few areas, research findings also differed from previous research findings and the recommendations in the framing guide:

◆ Participants desired attention-getting information at the beginning of the messages. Because the concept frame is a commonly-accepted cultural norm, this was not dramatic or attention-getting for many as a stand-alone message.

◆ Participants advocated for strong and dramatic language, but they did not identify with the examples of strong language statements from the framing guide.

◆ Participants did not like or understand a wide list of seemingly unrelated injury areas.

To incorporate these new findings into the existing coordinated messaging considerations, the following actions may be taken:

◆ The beginning of any message should use proven social marketing techniques to capture attention, such as strong statements and social math facts. Communicators should work to incorporate the concept frame throughout the entire message set.

◆ Wording connected to living to one's "full potential" should be stronger to capture audience members' attention. Language about the problem of injury and violence prevention should be stronger. Avoid general, nonspecific language in messages where appropriate.

◆ Because individuals have a hard time seeing how multiple injuries and violence are related, messages that list multiple injury topics should include more language to highlight the connection. As communicators continue to reference multiple types of injury and violence topics, audiences can better understand the types of health problems related to injury and violence as a field. For specific contexts where the listing of multiple injury might be too distracting, communicators may also consider connecting their specific injury issue to a larger statement about injury overall.

A few additional message characteristics were also important:

◆ Participants identified most strongly with the concept frame of "full potential" when expressed in language that resonated with them (e.g., older adults identify more with the words "quality of life" as full potential and parents identify more with "full potential" when messages concern their children).

◆ Messages should focus on the preventability of injury as individuals still don't see how injuries are preventable, particularly ones resulting from violence.

◆ Messages should help audience members to identify with how particular injuries may affect them or their loved ones.

The SSNR frame was perceived positively and similarly to the full potential frame—both frames can be integrated into violence prevention and response messages for cohesive communication.

Appendix B
Steps for Creating Social Math[8]

Steps for Creating Social Math

1. Consider the Frame
Look at the selected frame and the research supporting it, and review the message testing research culminating in the final message. This is the main focus when developing the social math, so keep this frame in mind throughout. The frame we've developed for those who work in the field of injury is—"we want a society where people can live to their full potential."

To incorporate social math successfully into an overall communication strategy, look at what the research says the frame needs to accomplish. Social math can then help set a new frame by:

◆ Connecting two or more things together

◆ Comparing the size of things

◆ Functioning as a metaphor.

2. Consider Relevant Injury Examples
Consider specific, relevant injury examples that will resonate with the public and the media. Consider using injury issues, such as children's bicycle helmets, teenagers' drinking and driving incidents, child abuse and neglect, traumatic brain injury, falls among older adults, or motor vehicle crashes, which clearly reflect the value of the frame.

3. Consider Relevant Statistics for the Injury Issues[9]
It is critical that you select numbers that best support your goal and those that would be compelling. Keep the overall number of statistics you use in interviews, graphs, and other media-related materials to a minimum. Also use statistics in slide presentations, briefings, town meetings, podcasts, and other communication vehicles.

---

[8] The social math message examples provided in this section are for illustrative purposes only. The messages have not been tested with members of the intended audience nor pre-screened and cleared by NCIPC. Prior to using these messages, it is recommended that you pre-test the messages with members of your target audience.

[9] Dorfman, L., Woodruff, K., Herbert, K., & Ervice, J. (2004). *Making the case for early care and education: A message development guide for advocates* (pp. 112-114). Berkeley, CA: Berkeley Media Studies Group. Available at: http://www.bmsg.org/documents/YellowBookrev.pdf.

Begin by selecting 5 to 10 key statistics that are related to the point you are trying to prove. As you will see below, these could be about the number of injuries, morbidity, mortality, funding, personnel or time spent on the issue, or almost anything as long as it relates back to the frame. Begin by focusing on the numbers of people, injuries, fatalities, or hours, rather than percentages, which can be more difficult to translate into social math.

◆ *Break the numbers down by time.*

If you know the amount over a year, what does that look like per hour? Per minute? For example, the average annual salary of a childcare worker nationally is $15,430, roughly $7.42 per hour. While many people understand that an annual salary of $15,430 is low, breaking the figure down by the hour reinforces that point—and makes the need for some kind of intervention even more clear.

◆ *Break down the numbers by place.*

Comparing a statistic with a well-known place can give people a sense of the statistic's magnitude. For instance, approximately 250,000 children are on waiting lists for childcare subsidies in California. That's enough children to fill almost every seat in every Major League ballpark in California. Such a comparison helps us visualize the scope of the problem and makes a solution all the more imperative.

◆ *Provide comparisons with familiar things.*

Providing a comparison to something that is familiar can have great impact. For example, "While Head Start is a successful, celebrated educational program, it is so underfunded that it serves only about three-fifths of eligible children. Applying that proportion to social security would mean that almost a million currently eligible seniors wouldn't receive benefits."

◆ *Provide ironic comparisons.*

For example, the average annual cost of full-time, licensed, center-based care for a child under age 2 in California is twice the tuition at the University of California at Berkeley. What's ironic here is how out of balance our public conversation is. Parents and the public focus so much on the cost of college when earlier education is dramatically more expensive.

◆ *Localize the numbers.*

Make comparisons that will resonate with community members. For example, saying, "Center-based childcare for an infant costs $11,450 per year in Seattle, Washington," is one thing. Saying, "In Seattle, Washington, a father making minimum wage would have to spend 79 percent of his income per year to place his baby in a licensed care center," is much more powerful because it illustrates why it is nearly impossible.

4. Finding Useful Comparison Statistics

Once you have an idea of what you want to say and how you want to say it, you will need to complete the cycle by filling in useful comparisons from outside the field of injury research. Avoid controversial topics for your comparison, including politics, crime, other health issues, or anything that could get twisted out of context. For example, one way to highlight a large amount of money is to compare it with the amount currently being spent on your issue.

5. Fact Checking and Polishing for Presentation

Put all the pieces together in a simple, seamless statement, which clearly demonstrates your position. Double check the statistics for the comparison data. Have the data and formulas you used available for reference when presenting the social math examples.

Run your social math example by colleagues to make sure it is clear, compelling, and unoffensive. Ensure that your numbers have a strong scientific basis and do not detract from your point or damage your credibility. Pay careful attention to the accuracy of the claims you are making. If you are using math for advocacy, you must be able to understand and defend the data and the way you are presenting the information.

Five Lessons for Using Numbers More Effectively

1. Unless numbers are married to a story, they are unlikely to mean anything to the public.

◆   Provide the meaning first and then use the numbers to support that meaning.

◆   What is the organizing principle or frame that the numbers support?

2. Too often, numbers are used to tell one story—crisis.

◆   The crisis frame incapacitates people and does not engage them in fixing the problem.

◆   Often the crisis frame describing a big problem is followed with a small solution, which seems meaningless or futile.

◆   Ask instead, "What is the story that our numbers could be used to tell that allows people to see solutions?" Think "David and Goliath" (little triumphing over large) or the "Little Engine that Could" (succeeding in the face of great adversity).

3. Social math unifies the narrative and the numbers.

◆   Provide the framing cues that are missing in the raw numbers. For example, "Community residents near a gasoline refinery noted that the plant emits 6 tons of pollutants per day— or 25 balloons full of toxic pollution for each school child in the town."

◆ By explaining one number in terms of another, the problem gets defined—pollutants (the issue) are "about" health and what's at stake is our children (advocacy).

◆ Make sure you choose the right value for your comparison (can backfire otherwise). For example, "Americans spend more on pet food than on helmets and body protection equipment."

4. Use numbers to support causal stories.

◆ Outline the story your numbers need to support as a chain of events in which the influences of each are apparent. For example, "Sea levels rise because our cars are pumping more carbon dioxide into the air, fish die in the oceans, and the food chain is disrupted. Here are the facts [insert math facts and statistics to support your statements above]. And here's how it could work differently."

◆ Simple causal sequences are important in helping people understand context, human impacts, prevention, and the efficacy of solutions.

5. Uninterpreted numbers tell a story of random mayhem.

◆ Random mayhem means that there is no room for human causality, prevention, or government responsibility.

◆ Use numbers to describe what could have been done to prevent the problem.

◆ Relating just the facts or the numbers does not inspire obligation from your reader to take action.

Social Math Examples

These injury-specific social math facts were developed by CDC's National Center for Injury Prevention and Control Division of Injury Response:

Acute Care

◆ "Each year, U.S. emergency departments treat more than 30 million nonfatal injuries. That is more than the populations of Montana, Nevada, New Mexico, and Texas combined."

◆ "If you are severely injured, getting care at a Level I trauma center can reduce your risk of death by 25 percent. For every 100,000 people who are severely injured, 2400 lives can be saved."

Traumatic Brain Injury

◆ "As many as 3.8 million sports- and recreation-related concussions occur each year in the United States. That's enough people to fill the 2008 super bowl stadium more than 50 times." (University of Phoenix Stadium capacity is 73,719.)

   ▫ Or, "That's equal to the current population of Oregon."

   ▫ Or, "That's equal to the current population of Los Angeles."

◆ "More than 1.6 million people are seen in an emergency department, are hospitalized, or die from a traumatic brain injury in the United States each year. That's more than the number of people who live in the cities of Baltimore, MD, Washington, DC, and Richmond, VA combined."

Alcohol Screening and Brief Intervention

◆ "In the United States, the third leading cause of preventable death and the leading risk factor for serious injury is alcohol misuse. It accounts for more than 75,000 deaths annually—one death every 7 minutes."

These injury-specific social math facts were developed by CDC's National Center for Injury Prevention and Control, Division of Unintentional Injury Prevention:

Falls Prevention

◆ "Based on 2006 mortality data, every 35 minutes an older adult dies from a fall-related injury."

◆ "Every day 5,000 adults age 65 and above are hospitalized due to fall-related injuries."

◆ "In 2008, falls accounted for 64% or 2.1 million nonfatal injuries treated in emergency departments. In other words, every 15 seconds, an older adult was treated in an emergency department for a fall."

Motor Vehicle Injury Prevention

◆ "Every 15 minutes, a 16- to 19-year-old teen is admitted to an emergency department because of motor vehicle crash-related injuries."

◆ "Every day, an average of 12 teenagers between ages 16 and 19 die as a result of a motor vehicle crash."

◆ "Only 1 in 10 teens buckles up when riding in a vehicle with someone else. Teenagers' passengers are less likely to wear their safety belts than any other age group."

Fire Injury Prevention

◆ "People who don't have working smoke alarms in their homes are twice as likely to die in a fire than those with working alarms."

These violence-specific social math facts were developed by CDC's National Center for Injury Prevention and Control, Division of Violence Prevention:

Violence Prevention

◆ "Nationwide implementation of effective school-based programs to prevent youth violence could result in 187,000 fewer fight-related injuries among high school students. That's equivalent to nearly 7,500 classrooms of students."

◆ "Over 5 percent of high school students report missing school at least once in the past 30 days because of safety concerns. This is the equivalent of approximately 25,000 classrooms of high school students missing school because of fear."

◆ "Each year over 91,000 infants less than 1 year old are victims of substantiated child maltreatment. If we were to place these infants' cribs end-to-end, the line of cribs would stretch for 78 miles."

◆ "The number of homicide victims in the United States each year could fill 32 Boeing 747 airplanes. Can you imagine how much concern there would be if 32 airplanes fell out of the sky in the U.S. in a given year?"

◆ "If all low- income families in the United States received nurse home visitation services, 300,000 cases of child maltreatment could be prevented each year."

◆ "There are over 32,000 suicides each year in the United States—this means that there is a suicide every 16 minutes."

The following are general social math facts:

◆ "In 1969, for many students, walking to school was as easy as walking down the street because their school was in their neighborhood. By 2001, most schools were farther away from their students, and walking or biking to school was the equivalent of doing a 5K race or more— twice a day."

◆ "Exercise is something that children need every day, but half of all students attend schools that have reduced their physical education class to just 1 or 2 days per week. Part-time fitness is no more effective than part-time reading or math instruction."

◆ "Coca-Cola and Pepsi alone spend 100 times more on advertising than the Federal *Fruits & Veggies—More Matters* healthy diet campaign."

◆ "Between 1971 and 2002, the Trust for Public Land's work in cities resulted in the acquisition of 532 properties totaling 40,754 acres. That's like adding park space equivalent to 326,000 soccer fields. What a terrific opportunity to engage in healthy activities that influence one's full potential."

◆ "In 1991, U.S. college students consumed 430 million gallons of alcoholic beverages per year at a cost of $5.5 billion. Enough alcohol was consumed by college students to fill 3,500 Olympic-size swimming pools, about one on every campus in the United States."

◆ "In 1991, U.S. college students consumed 430 million gallons of alcoholic beverages per year at a cost of $5.5 billion. The overall amount spent on alcohol per student exceeded the dollars spent on books and was far greater than the combined amount of fellowships and scholarships provided to students."

◆ "The alcohol industry spends more than $2 billion every year to advertise and promote consumption. This amounts to approximately $225,000 every hour of every day."

◆ "Health benefit costs of the employees who build tractors costs more than the steel that goes into a tractor."

Sources

Social Math Fact Sources

◆ Center for Health Improvement
http://www.chipolicy.org/pdf/TA5.pdf

◆ Department of Community Medicine, University of Connecticut Health Center
http://www.commed.uchc.edu/healthservices/mediaadvoc/sld001.htm

◆ InfoPlease
http://www.infoplease.com/us.html

◆ Census Bureau Quick Facts
http://quickfacts.census.gov/qfd/index.html

◆ FrameWorks Example of "How-To"
http://www.frameworksinstitute.org/ezine39.html
http://www.frameworksinstitute.org/ezine40.html

◆ Table 1 on Page 8
Adapted from the NCIPC Injury Communication Planning Tools
National Center for Injury Prevention and Control
Centers for Disease Control and Prevention
January 2007

Injury Framing Tool sources

◆ *Traumatic Brain Injury*
Rutland-Brown, W., Langlois. J. A., Thomas, K. E., Xi, Y. L. (2006). *Incidence of traumatic brain injury in the United States, 2003. Journal of Head Trauma Rehabilitation, 21*, 544-548.

◆ Langlois, J. A., Rutland-Brown, W., Wald, M. (2006). *The epidemiology and impact of traumatic brain injury: A brief overview. Journal of Head Trauma Rehabilitation, 21*(5), 375-378.

◆ *Field Triage.*
MacKenzie, E. J., Rivara, P., Jurkovich, G., et al. (2006). *A national evaluation of the effort of trauma-center care on mortality. New England Journal of Medicine, 354(4):366-378.*

◆ *Older Adult Falls*
Grisso, J. A., Kelsey, J. L., Strom, B. L., Chiu, G. Y., Maislin, G., O'Brien, L. A., et al. (1991). *Risk factors for falls as a cause of hip fracture in women: The Northeast Hip Fracture Study Group. New England Journal of Medicine, 324(19):1326–1331.*

◆ *Fire Prevention*
National Fire Protection Association
http://www.nfpa.org/categoryList.asp?categoryID=278&URL=
Research%2&%20Reports/Fact%20sheets/Smoke%20alarms

◆ *Intimate Partner Violence Prevention*
U.S Department of Justice
http://www.ojp.usdoj.gov/bjs/homicide/intimates.htm

◆ *Youth Violence Prevention*
Centers for Disease Control and Prevention
http://www.cdc.gov/ncipc/dvp/YVP/YVP-data.htm

◆ *Child Abuse and Neglect*
http://www.cdc.gov/ncipc/pub-res/parenting/ChildMalT-Briefing.pdf
http://www.cdc.gov/ncipc/dvp/CMP/child_maltreatment.htm

Appendix C
Formative Research

The frame developed for this publication was created from discussions with injury communication professionals and was tested through focus groups with members of the public. CDC's Injury Center sought to identify an overarching message frame that individuals and organizations involved in injury and violence prevention and response would be willing to use and that would also resonate with the public.

In focus groups conducted by CDC's Injury Center and the Hawaii State Department of Health, members of the public reviewed and provided feedback on the messages. The groups were intended to identify the frame that would have the greatest impact and the messages that would support the frame. These focus groups offered the opportunity to see and hear the immediate reactions to the proposed messages and then probe for reasons behind these reactions. We listened carefully to the thoughts, opinions, and experiences of the participants, which, in turn, provided insight into how the messages would be received and ultimately how they might motivate behavior change or action.

CDC's Injury Center believes more research is needed with members of the public to provide a greater depth of understanding about how this message frame can be used effectively across the breadth of injury and violence prevention issues. Those interested in conducting focus groups should consider the guidelines described below.

Recruitment of participants will require development of eligibility criteria and a recruitment screener. It may be that focus group participants should reflect the general population so that the screening results in participants who represent a broad spectrum of racial and ethnic populations and educational and income levels. Research that focuses on audiences susceptible to, or particularly concerned with, an area of injury or violence prevention will also be important.

The moderator guide should include a variety of open-ended questions that explore reactions to the frame and the messages being tested. The questions below provide examples of the type of information you are trying to gather:

◆ What does this message mean to you?

◆ What is clear or unclear about this message?

◆ Tell me how this message gets you to think more about injuries and how they can be prevented and responded to. What part specifically?

◆ How well do you think these different messages convey the value statement of wanting to live in a society where people can live to their full potential?

◆ Which one of the messages elicits the greatest emotional reaction?

◆ Tell me about the message you prefer.

◆ Tell me about the message, if any, you dislike?

◆ Tell me about the part of the message you can relate to the most.

◆ Tell me about how the message makes you want to get involved in doing something about injury in your community or in your home. Which parts specifically?

◆ This message suggests different benefits of living in a society where individuals can live to their full potential. Which message provides the most valuable benefit to you? To your community?

To take full advantage of the opportunity to hear from participants, a professionally trained moderator and a note taker should be engaged for each group. Focus groups should be audio-recorded and, if possible, transcribed so researchers can review the actual words spoken in their analysis of themes and development of findings.

So that everyone working to develop coordinated messages on injury and violence prevention and response can improve communication, researchers are encouraged to share their findings.

U.S. Department of Health and Human Services
Centers for Disease Control and Prevention
National Center for Injury Prevention and Control
www.cdc.gov/Injury

We Want a Society Where People Can Live to Their Full Potential.